Copyright © 2023 by Lily J. Thompson (Author)

This book is protected by copyright law and is intended solely for personal use. Reproduction, distribution, or any other form of use requires the written permission of the author. The information presented in this book is for educational and entertainment purposes only, and while every effort has been made to ensure its accuracy and completeness, no guarantees are made. The author is not providing legal, financial, medical, or professional advice, and readers should consult with a licensed professional before implementing any of the techniques discussed in this book. The content in this book has been sourced from various reliable sources, but readers should exercise their own judgment when using this information. The author is not responsible for any losses, direct or indirect, that may occur from the use of this book, including but not limited to errors, omissions, or inaccuracies.

We hope this book has been informative and helpful on your journey to understanding and celebrating older adults. Thank you for your interest and support!

Title: The Joy of Upcycling
Subtitle: A Minimalist's Guide to Creatively Reducing Waste and Saving Resources

Series: The Joy of Less: A Minimalist's Guide to Happiness
By Lily J. Thompson

"Minimalism is not a lack of something. It's simply the perfect amount of something."

Nicholas Burroughs

"Minimalism is not a style, it is an attitude, a way of being. It's a fundamental reaction against noise, visual noise, disorder, vulgarity. Minimalism is the pursuit of the essence of things, not the appearance."

Claudio Silvestrin

"Minimalism is the intentional promotion of the things we most value and the removal of anything that distracts us from it."

Joshua Becker

"Simplicity is the ultimate sophistication."

Leonardo da Vinci

"The ability to simplify means to eliminate the unnecessary so that the necessary may speak."

Hans Hofmann

"Minimalism is not a lack of personality, it's a matter of emphasizing what's important."

Unknown

"Minimalism is not about living in a stark, empty space. It's about surrounding yourself with the things you love and use most often."

Unknown

Table of Contents

Introduction
The Impact of Consumerism on the Environment

Consumerism is a driving force of modern society. It promotes the idea that more is better, and that we should constantly seek to accumulate more material goods, regardless of their quality or necessity. However, this mentality comes at a cost. Our planet is facing unprecedented environmental challenges, including climate change, biodiversity loss, and pollution. Many of these issues can be traced back to our consumerist culture, which prioritizes economic growth and individual consumption over environmental sustainability and social justice.

The Environmental Cost of Consumerism

One of the main impacts of consumerism on the environment is the overuse of natural resources. Our demand for products and services requires the extraction of materials such as timber, minerals, and fossil fuels at an unsustainable rate. This leads to deforestation, soil erosion, and water scarcity, as well as the depletion of non-renewable resources such as oil and gas. In addition, the production and disposal of goods generate large amounts of waste and emissions, contributing to air and water pollution, greenhouse gas emissions, and climate change.

The Social Cost of Consumerism

Consumerism also has social consequences, particularly for marginalized communities and future generations. The pursuit of economic growth often comes at the expense of human rights, as corporations prioritize profits over workers' rights, public health, and social welfare. The production of goods can also have negative impacts on the health and well-being of local communities, particularly in developing countries where environmental regulations are weak. In addition, the accumulation of debt and the pressure to consume can lead to stress, anxiety, and social isolation, further exacerbating the negative impact of consumerism on mental health and social cohesion.

Alternative Models of Consumption

Given the environmental and social costs of consumerism, it is essential to explore alternative models of consumption that prioritize sustainability, equity, and well-being. One such model is minimalism, which promotes living with less and reducing waste. By consuming mindfully and intentionally, we can reduce our ecological footprint and live a more meaningful and fulfilling life. Other models include the circular economy, which seeks to minimize waste and maximize the use of resources through reuse, repair, and recycling, and the sharing economy, which encourages the sharing of goods and services to reduce overconsumption and increase community resilience.

Conclusion

The impact of consumerism on the environment is undeniable. Our current economic model is not sustainable, and urgent action is needed to shift towards more environmentally and socially responsible modes of consumption. By reducing our reliance on material goods, and embracing more sustainable and equitable models of consumption, we can create a better future for ourselves and for the planet.

The Benefits of Minimalist Materials

Minimalism is a lifestyle philosophy that advocates for living with less, and reducing clutter and waste. It has gained popularity in recent years as a response to our consumerist culture and its impact on the environment and personal well-being. Minimalism promotes a shift towards more intentional and sustainable consumption, focusing on quality over quantity, and reducing our reliance on material possessions. In this section, we will explore the benefits of minimalist materials for the environment, personal well-being, and social justice.

The Environmental Benefits of Minimalist Materials

One of the main benefits of minimalist materials is their positive impact on the environment. By consuming less and reducing waste, we can reduce our ecological footprint and contribute to a more sustainable future. Minimalism promotes the use of natural and sustainable materials, which are less harmful to the environment than synthetic materials such as plastic or polyester. By investing in quality and long-lasting products, we can reduce the need for constant replacement and disposal, which in turn reduces waste and emissions. Additionally, minimalist materials often prioritize energy efficiency and resource conservation, leading to a further reduction in environmental impact.

The Personal Benefits of Minimalist Materials

In addition to the environmental benefits, minimalist materials also have numerous personal benefits. By living with less, we can reduce clutter and create a more peaceful and organized living space. This can lead to a reduction in stress and anxiety, and an increase in mental clarity and creativity. Minimalism also promotes a more intentional and mindful approach to consumption, leading to a deeper appreciation for the things we do have, and a reduction in the pressure to constantly consume more. This can lead to a greater sense of personal satisfaction and fulfillment.

The Social Benefits of Minimalist Materials

Minimalism also has social benefits, particularly in terms of social justice and equity. By reducing our consumption and waste, we can reduce the negative impact of overconsumption on marginalized communities and future generations. Additionally, by prioritizing sustainable and ethical products, we can support local and fair trade practices, and reduce the negative impact of globalized supply chains on workers' rights and public health. Finally, minimalist materials can promote a sense of community and shared values, as we connect with others who share our commitment to sustainability and intentional living.

Conclusion

Minimalist materials offer numerous benefits for the environment, personal well-being, and social justice. By reducing our reliance on material possessions, and embracing a more intentional and sustainable approach to consumption, we can create a more fulfilling and meaningful life, while also contributing to a more just and sustainable future for ourselves and for the planet.

How to Adopt a Minimalist Materials Lifestyle

Adopting a minimalist materials lifestyle is a journey that involves a shift in mindset, habits, and values. It requires us to question our assumptions about what we need to be happy, and to re-evaluate our relationship with material possessions and the environment. In this section, we will explore practical strategies and tips for adopting a minimalist materials lifestyle, including decluttering, reducing waste, and embracing sustainable and ethical consumption.

Decluttering Your Home

The first step towards a minimalist materials lifestyle is decluttering your home. This involves evaluating your possessions and letting go of items that no longer serve a purpose or bring you joy. There are several strategies for decluttering, including the KonMari method, which involves organizing your possessions by category and only keeping items that "spark joy." Another strategy is the "one in, one out" rule, which involves getting rid of one item for every new item you bring into your home. The goal of decluttering is to create a living space that is clean, organized, and free of unnecessary clutter, which can help reduce stress and improve mental clarity.

Reducing Waste

Another important aspect of a minimalist materials lifestyle is reducing waste. This involves adopting a "zero waste" or "low waste" mindset, and making choices that prioritize sustainable and ethical consumption. Some practical strategies for reducing waste include:

- Refusing single-use plastic items such as straws, water bottles, and bags.

- Recycling and composting to reduce the amount of waste sent to landfills.

- Choosing products with minimal packaging or packaging that is recyclable or compostable.

- Repairing and repurposing items rather than replacing them.

- Investing in quality and long-lasting products that are less likely to need replacement.

Sustainable and Ethical Consumption

Finally, a minimalist materials lifestyle involves embracing sustainable and ethical consumption. This involves making choices that prioritize the environment, social justice, and fair trade practices. Some practical strategies for sustainable and ethical consumption include:

- Choosing natural and sustainable materials such as organic cotton, bamboo, or linen.

- Supporting local and fair trade businesses and products.

- Researching brands and products to ensure they align with your values.

- Embracing a "less is more" mindset and prioritizing quality over quantity.

- Choosing products that are energy-efficient and resource-conserving.

Conclusion

Adopting a minimalist materials lifestyle requires a shift in mindset, habits, and values. It involves decluttering your home, reducing waste, and embracing sustainable and ethical consumption. By adopting these practices, we can create a more intentional and fulfilling life, while also contributing to a more just and sustainable future for ourselves and for the planet.

Chapter 1: Understanding Minimalism and Sustainability

Defining Minimalism and Sustainability

Minimalism and sustainability are two concepts that have gained significant attention in recent years due to their potential to help address issues related to consumerism, materialism, and environmental degradation. While these terms are often used interchangeably, they have distinct definitions and implications.

Minimalism refers to a lifestyle characterized by intentional living, simplicity, and the elimination of excess possessions and distractions. It involves a conscious choice to live with less, and to focus on what truly matters in life. Minimalists prioritize experiences, relationships, and personal growth over material possessions.

Sustainability, on the other hand, refers to the ability to meet the needs of the present without compromising the ability of future generations to meet their own needs. It is about creating a balance between economic development, social well-being, and environmental protection. Sustainable practices seek to minimize negative impacts on the planet and promote the long-term health and well-being of all living beings.

While minimalism and sustainability have different definitions, they share many similarities and are often intertwined. Minimalism can be seen as a means to achieve sustainability by reducing consumption, waste, and environmental impact. By choosing to live with less, minimalists often have a smaller environmental footprint and contribute less to consumerism and materialism.

Additionally, sustainability can be seen as a way to support a minimalist lifestyle by promoting ethical and responsible consumption. Sustainable products and practices align with the values of minimalism by prioritizing quality, durability, and longevity over disposability and excess.

In summary, while minimalism and sustainability have different definitions, they are complementary concepts that can support each other in creating a more intentional, responsible, and environmentally conscious way of living. By adopting a minimalist and sustainable lifestyle, individuals can contribute to a healthier planet, a more equitable society, and a more fulfilling life.

The Benefits of Minimalist Living for the Environment

Minimalist living has many benefits for the environment. By choosing to live with less, individuals can significantly reduce their environmental impact and contribute to a healthier planet. Here are some of the key ways in which minimalist living benefits the environment:

1. Reducing consumption: Minimalists prioritize the things that matter most to them, which often means consuming less overall. By reducing consumption, minimalists help to reduce the demand for new products and resources, which in turn reduces the amount of waste and pollution generated by the manufacturing and transportation of those products.

2. Minimizing waste: Minimalists are often mindful of the waste they produce and strive to minimize it as much as possible. This can involve practices such as composting, recycling, and upcycling, as well as avoiding single-use items and unnecessary packaging. By minimizing waste, minimalists help to reduce the amount of waste that ends up in landfills, oceans, and other natural environments.

3. Lowering carbon footprint: Minimalists often choose to live in smaller spaces, which require less energy to heat and cool. They may also choose to live in walkable

neighborhoods, use public transportation, or opt for fuel-efficient vehicles. By lowering their carbon footprint, minimalists help to reduce greenhouse gas emissions and combat climate change.

4. Supporting sustainable products and practices: Minimalists often prioritize quality over quantity and choose products that are sustainably produced and ethically sourced. This can include products made from natural and renewable materials, as well as those that are manufactured using environmentally friendly processes. By supporting sustainable products and practices, minimalists help to promote responsible and ethical consumption.

5. Encouraging a shift towards a circular economy: Minimalists often embrace the concept of a circular economy, in which resources are used and reused in a closed loop. This involves practices such as upcycling, repairing, and sharing resources, as well as minimizing waste and pollution. By encouraging a shift towards a circular economy, minimalists help to reduce resource depletion and promote a more sustainable way of life.

In conclusion, minimalist living offers many benefits for the environment. By reducing consumption, minimizing waste, lowering their carbon footprint, supporting sustainable products and practices, and encouraging a shift towards a circular economy, minimalists can help to create a healthier and more sustainable planet. By adopting a minimalist lifestyle, individuals can make a positive impact on the environment and contribute to a more sustainable future for all.

The Importance of Sustainable Consumption

Sustainable consumption refers to the use of goods and services that minimize environmental impact and preserve natural resources for future generations. It is a crucial aspect of sustainable living and an essential component of a minimalist materials lifestyle. In this section, we will discuss the importance of sustainable consumption and how it can positively impact the environment.

1. Preserves Natural Resources

Sustainable consumption is critical in preserving natural resources, such as water, land, and forests. By consuming products that are made sustainably, we can reduce the amount of waste and pollution that results from traditional manufacturing processes. Additionally, we can reduce the demand for raw materials and energy required to produce these products, ultimately preserving natural resources for future generations.

2. Reduces Waste

Sustainable consumption helps to reduce waste by using products that are designed to be reused, recycled, or composted. These products are typically made from sustainable materials, such as bamboo, recycled plastic, or biodegradable materials, and are designed to minimize waste at every stage of their lifecycle. By reducing waste, we can also reduce the amount of pollution that is released into the environment, including greenhouse gas emissions that contribute to climate change.

3. Supports Ethical Practices

Sustainable consumption also supports ethical practices, such as fair trade, which ensures that workers are treated fairly and paid a living wage. It also encourages companies to adopt environmentally friendly practices, such as reducing their carbon footprint and using renewable energy sources. By supporting companies that prioritize sustainability and ethical practices, we can help to create a more just and equitable world.

4. Promotes Health and Well-Being

Sustainable consumption can also promote health and well-being by encouraging us to adopt healthier and more sustainable lifestyles. By consuming organic, locally grown produce, for example, we can reduce our exposure to harmful pesticides and support local farmers. By reducing our consumption of processed foods and animal products, we can also improve our overall health and reduce the risk of chronic diseases.

5. Empowers Consumers

Sustainable consumption also empowers consumers to make informed choices about the products they buy and the companies they support. By educating ourselves about the environmental and social impact of the products we consume, we can make more conscious choices that align with our values and beliefs. This can ultimately create a more sustainable and equitable society.

In conclusion, sustainable consumption is a critical component of a minimalist materials lifestyle and an essential aspect of creating a more sustainable and just world. By consuming products that preserve natural resources, reduce waste, support ethical practices, promote health and well-being, and empower consumers, we can make a positive impact on the environment and create a brighter future for generations to come.

The Impact of Fast Fashion on the Environment

Fast fashion has become a major issue when it comes to sustainability. Fast fashion is a term used to describe a quick and inexpensive approach to clothing production. It involves the rapid design, production, and sale of clothing items that are meant to be worn only a few times before being discarded. The fast fashion industry has been able to produce a vast quantity of clothing items at low costs, making it accessible to the mass market. However, this production model comes at a high cost to the environment.

Environmental Impact of Fast Fashion

The fast fashion industry has a significant impact on the environment, from the production of raw materials to the disposal of the final product. Here are some of the ways in which fast fashion impacts the environment:

1. Overproduction and waste: Fast fashion companies produce large quantities of clothing that often end up unsold or discarded. This results in a significant amount of waste and pollution.

2. Water consumption: The production of cotton, one of the most common materials used in clothing, requires vast amounts of water. The production of one cotton t-shirt can require up to 2,700 liters of water, according to the World Wildlife Fund.

3. Chemicals and pollution: The fast fashion industry uses a range of chemicals in its production process, including dyes, bleaches, and finishing agents. These chemicals can have harmful effects on both the environment and human health. Additionally, the disposal of these chemicals can lead to water pollution.

4. Carbon emissions: The fast fashion industry is responsible for a significant amount of carbon emissions. According to the United Nations, the fashion industry is responsible for 10% of global carbon emissions.

5. Working conditions: The fast fashion industry is known for its poor working conditions and low wages for workers in developing countries. This not only impacts the workers but also the environment as the lack of regulations can lead to environmental damage.

Sustainable Alternatives to Fast Fashion

There are several sustainable alternatives to fast fashion that can help reduce the environmental impact of clothing production. Here are some examples:

1. Sustainable materials: Clothing made from sustainable materials, such as organic cotton, hemp, and bamboo, can help reduce the environmental impact of clothing production.

2. Second-hand clothing: Purchasing second-hand clothing is an excellent way to reduce the environmental impact of clothing production. It keeps clothing out of landfills and reduces the demand for new clothing.

3. Slow fashion: Slow fashion focuses on producing high-quality, long-lasting clothing items that are meant to be worn for years, rather than just a few times.

4. Ethical and sustainable brands: Many clothing brands are committed to sustainable and ethical production methods. These brands often use sustainable materials, reduce waste, and provide fair wages and safe working conditions for their workers.

Conclusion

The fast fashion industry has a significant impact on the environment, from overproduction and waste to pollution and carbon emissions. Sustainable alternatives, such as second-hand clothing, slow fashion, and ethical and sustainable brands, can help reduce the environmental impact of clothing production. It is important to make informed decisions when it comes to clothing consumption and support sustainable and ethical practices in the fashion industry.

Chapter 2: Reducing Waste in Your Home
The Problem with Single-Use Plastics

Single-use plastics are designed for one-time use before being disposed of. They are widely used in packaging, food service, and retail industries, and their convenience and low cost have made them a popular choice for consumers. However, the environmental impact of single-use plastics is significant.

Plastic is a non-biodegradable material, meaning that it does not break down naturally in the environment. When single-use plastics are not properly disposed of, they end up in landfills, littering the streets, or polluting waterways. According to a report by the United Nations, over 8 million tons of plastic enter the oceans every year, threatening marine life and ecosystems.

Single-use plastics have become a major contributor to plastic pollution, with plastic bags, straws, and food packaging being the most commonly found items in the environment. Plastic bags, for example, can take up to 1,000 years to decompose, and during that time, they can release harmful chemicals and microplastics that contaminate the soil and water.

In addition to their environmental impact, single-use plastics also have economic consequences. The cost of managing plastic waste is estimated to be $40 billion a year globally, and the cost is projected to increase to $75 billion by 2030 if current trends continue. This cost includes the collection, transportation, and disposal of plastic waste, as well as the damage caused by plastic pollution to fisheries, tourism, and other industries.

To address the problem of single-use plastics, individuals and businesses can take several actions. One of the most effective ways to reduce plastic waste is to refuse single-use plastics altogether. Consumers can bring their reusable bags, bottles, and containers when shopping or eating out, and businesses can switch to reusable or compostable alternatives. Governments can also implement policies to ban or tax single-use plastics and promote sustainable alternatives.

In conclusion, the problem with single-use plastics is a significant environmental and economic challenge. The use of single-use plastics contributes to plastic pollution, which harms the environment and threatens marine life. Reducing our reliance on single-use plastics through sustainable consumption habits and policy changes is essential to creating a more sustainable future.

Reducing Waste through Recycling and Upcycling

Reducing waste through recycling and upcycling is one of the key ways in which we can reduce our environmental impact and live more sustainably. Recycling and upcycling help to conserve natural resources, reduce landfill waste, and decrease greenhouse gas emissions. In this section, we will explore the benefits of recycling and upcycling, as well as some tips and strategies for incorporating these practices into your daily life.

Benefits of Recycling

Recycling is the process of converting waste materials into new products, thereby reducing the need for virgin materials and conserving natural resources. The benefits of recycling are numerous and include:

1. Conserving Natural Resources: Recycling reduces the need for raw materials, such as timber, minerals, and petroleum, which are used to make new products. By using recycled materials, we can conserve these natural resources and reduce the environmental impact associated with their extraction and processing.

2. Reducing Energy Consumption: The production of new products requires energy, which contributes to greenhouse gas emissions and other environmental impacts. By recycling materials, we can reduce the energy required to

produce new products, thereby decreasing greenhouse gas emissions and other environmental impacts.

3. Reducing Landfill Waste: Recycling helps to reduce the amount of waste sent to landfills, which can have a range of environmental impacts. Landfills can generate methane gas, a potent greenhouse gas, as well as leachate, which can contaminate soil and water resources. By recycling materials, we can reduce the amount of waste sent to landfills and minimize these impacts.

Tips for Recycling

Here are some tips for incorporating recycling into your daily life:

1. Understand Your Local Recycling Program: Recycling programs vary from place to place, so it's important to understand what materials can be recycled in your area and how to properly prepare them for recycling.

2. Reduce Contamination: Contamination occurs when non-recyclable materials are mixed in with recyclable materials, making it difficult to separate and process the recyclable materials. To reduce contamination, make sure to clean and properly prepare your recyclables before placing them in the recycling bin.

3. Recycle Electronic Waste: Electronic waste, or e-waste, contains a range of toxic materials that can harm the

environment if not properly disposed of. Many communities have e-waste recycling programs, so make sure to properly dispose of your old electronics to minimize their environmental impact.

Benefits of Upcycling

Upcycling is the process of transforming waste materials into new products of higher value, quality, or environmental benefit. Upcycling helps to reduce waste, conserve resources, and minimize environmental impacts. The benefits of upcycling include:

1. Reducing Waste: Upcycling helps to reduce the amount of waste sent to landfills, thereby minimizing the environmental impacts associated with landfill waste.

2. Conserving Resources: Upcycling helps to conserve natural resources, such as timber, minerals, and petroleum, by reducing the need for virgin materials to produce new products.

3. Encouraging Creativity: Upcycling encourages creativity and innovation by challenging us to see waste materials as potential resources for new and innovative products.

Tips for Upcycling

Here are some tips for incorporating upcycling into your daily life:

1. Identify Potential Materials: Look for materials that can be upcycled, such as old clothing, furniture, and household items. Be creative and think outside the box!

2. Plan Your Projects: Before starting an upcycling project, plan out your design and materials to ensure a successful outcome.

3. Share Your Upcycling Successes: Share your upcycling successes with friends and family to inspire others to reduce waste and live more sustainably.

The Benefits of Composting

Composting is a natural process that transforms organic waste into nutrient-rich soil. It is an easy and effective way to reduce waste in your home and provide nutrient-rich soil for your plants. In this section, we will explore the benefits of composting and how you can start composting in your home.

1. Reducing Landfill Waste

When food waste and other organic materials are sent to a landfill, they produce methane, a potent greenhouse gas that contributes to climate change. Composting reduces the amount of organic waste that ends up in landfills, thereby reducing methane emissions.

2. Improving Soil Health

Compost is a nutrient-rich soil amendment that can improve soil health by adding organic matter, improving soil structure, and increasing nutrient availability. When you use compost in your garden, you are improving the health of your soil, which in turn supports healthy plant growth.

3. Reducing the Need for Chemical Fertilizers

Chemical fertilizers can have negative impacts on the environment, including contributing to water pollution and harming beneficial insects and other wildlife. Compost can provide many of the nutrients that plants need to grow without the need for chemical fertilizers.

4. Saving Money on Fertilizers and Soil Amendments

Compost is a cost-effective alternative to chemical fertilizers and other soil amendments. By composting at home, you can save money on these products and reduce your overall household expenses.

5. Supporting Biodiversity

Composting supports biodiversity by creating a healthy soil environment that supports a wide range of microorganisms, insects, and other wildlife. This diversity can support a healthy ecosystem and contribute to overall environmental health.

6. Closing the Nutrient Loop

Composting creates a closed loop system where organic waste is turned into nutrient-rich soil that can be used to grow new plants. This process reduces the need for external inputs and creates a sustainable system that supports long-term soil health and plant growth.

Overall, composting is an easy and effective way to reduce waste in your home and support a healthy environment. By composting at home, you can reduce landfill waste, improve soil health, save money, and support biodiversity.

Mindful Consumption of Products and Packaging

Mindful consumption of products and packaging is an essential aspect of reducing waste in your home. It involves being aware of the products and packaging you buy, using them mindfully, and disposing of them responsibly. Here are some ways to practice mindful consumption of products and packaging:

1. Avoid overconsumption: The first step towards mindful consumption is to avoid overconsumption. When you buy things you don't need or use excessively, you end up generating more waste. Hence, it is important to be mindful of what you buy and avoid unnecessary purchases.

2. Opt for sustainable products: Choose products made from sustainable materials, such as bamboo, glass, metal, or cloth. These materials are recyclable, reusable, and biodegradable, making them better choices for the environment.

3. Look for package-free options: Many products come with excessive packaging, which often ends up in the trash. Look for package-free options or products with minimal packaging to reduce waste.

4. Buy in bulk: Buying products in bulk reduces the amount of packaging needed per item, which reduces waste. Additionally, it can also save you money in the long run.

5. Use reusable bags: Using reusable bags instead of single-use plastic bags is a simple way to reduce waste. Keep a reusable bag with you at all times, so you don't need to rely on plastic bags when shopping.

6. Choose products with eco-friendly packaging: If you must buy products with packaging, choose ones with eco-friendly packaging, such as recycled paper or biodegradable materials.

7. Mindful disposal: When you are done using a product, dispose of it mindfully. Follow the recycling guidelines in your area, compost organic waste, and dispose of hazardous waste responsibly.

By practicing mindful consumption of products and packaging, you can reduce waste, save resources, and contribute to a more sustainable future. Additionally, it can also save you money in the long run and promote a simpler and more fulfilling lifestyle.

Chapter 3: Minimalist Materials for a Sustainable Home

Using Natural and Sustainable Materials

In today's world, it's essential to pay attention to the materials we use in our homes. Many common materials, such as plastic and synthetic materials, have a negative impact on the environment. Choosing natural and sustainable materials for your home can make a big difference in reducing your environmental footprint.

Natural materials are derived from natural sources such as plants, animals, and minerals. These materials are sustainable because they are renewable and biodegradable. They have a low environmental impact, and they often have health benefits over synthetic materials. Here are some examples of natural materials that you can use in your home:

1. Wood: Wood is a versatile material that can be used for many things in your home, such as furniture, flooring, and walls. It is a renewable resource, and if harvested responsibly, it can be a sustainable material. Wood is also biodegradable and has a low carbon footprint.

2. Bamboo: Bamboo is a fast-growing plant that is often used as an alternative to wood. It is a sustainable material because it grows quickly and requires fewer

resources to produce than wood. It can be used for flooring, furniture, and even textiles.

3. Cork: Cork is a renewable and biodegradable material that comes from the bark of cork trees. It is often used for flooring, wall tiles, and as a sustainable alternative to synthetic insulation.

4. Linoleum: Linoleum is a natural flooring material made from linseed oil, wood flour, and other natural materials. It is biodegradable and has a low carbon footprint. It is also durable and easy to maintain.

5. Stone: Natural stone, such as granite, marble, and slate, is a sustainable material that is often used for countertops, flooring, and walls. It is a durable and long-lasting material that is low-maintenance.

Sustainable materials are those that are produced using eco-friendly methods that have a low impact on the environment. These materials are often made from recycled materials, and they can be recycled again at the end of their life cycle. Here are some examples of sustainable materials that you can use in your home:

1. Recycled glass: Recycled glass is made from glass that has been collected and processed for reuse. It is often used for countertops, tiles, and decorative accents.

2. Recycled plastic: Recycled plastic is made from plastic that has been collected and processed for reuse. It can be used for a variety of products, including furniture, flooring, and building materials.

3. Hemp: Hemp is a sustainable material that is often used for textiles, such as rugs and curtains. It is a fast-growing plant that requires fewer resources to grow than cotton.

4. Wool: Wool is a natural and sustainable material that is often used for carpets and textiles. It is renewable, biodegradable, and has a low carbon footprint.

5. Reclaimed wood: Reclaimed wood is wood that has been salvaged from old buildings, pallets, or other sources. It is a sustainable material because it is reused instead of being discarded.

In conclusion, using natural and sustainable materials in your home is an essential step towards a more sustainable future. By choosing these materials, you can reduce your environmental footprint and enjoy the health benefits that come with using natural materials. It's important to do your research and choose materials that are both natural and sustainable, as not all natural materials are sustainable, and not all sustainable materials are natural.

Investing in Quality and Long-Lasting Products

Minimalism is not only about decluttering and simplifying your possessions; it's also about investing in high-quality, long-lasting products that will stand the test of time. In a consumerist culture that emphasizes disposability and planned obsolescence, this can be a significant shift in mindset. However, it is a vital step towards sustainable living and reducing waste.

Investing in quality products means purchasing items that are durable and well-made, with a focus on craftsmanship and longevity. When choosing products for your home, consider materials that are sustainable and environmentally friendly, such as natural fibers like linen, cotton, and wool, or materials that are recycled or upcycled.

One benefit of investing in quality products is that they often require less maintenance and repair, which can save you money in the long run. Cheaper, poorly made products may seem like a bargain at first, but they often need to be replaced more frequently, leading to higher costs over time. In contrast, high-quality products can last for years, even decades, with proper care.

Another benefit of investing in quality products is that they tend to be more functional and versatile. Instead of purchasing multiple items to perform different tasks, a single high-quality item may be able to fulfill multiple needs. For example, investing in a high-quality chef's knife can replace the need for several cheaper, lower-quality knives.

When considering which products to invest in, it's also essential to think about the values and ethics of the company that produces them. Look for companies that prioritize sustainability and ethical practices, such as fair labor standards and environmental responsibility. Supporting these companies sends a message that these values are important and helps promote positive change.

It's also important to remember that investing in quality products doesn't mean you need to spend a fortune. There are many affordable options for well-made, sustainable products. Consider purchasing from secondhand or vintage stores, or supporting small, independent businesses that prioritize sustainability and ethical practices.

In summary, investing in quality, long-lasting products is a crucial aspect of minimalist living and sustainable consumption. By choosing durable, sustainable, and versatile items, we can reduce waste, save money, and promote a more responsible and ethical consumer culture.

Sustainable Home Décor

Sustainable home decor refers to the practice of decorating your living space with environmentally conscious and socially responsible products. It is an integral part of a sustainable lifestyle that aims to minimize the negative impact of human activities on the planet.

Choosing sustainable home decor can be a daunting task, but it is essential to ensure that the products you use in your home do not contribute to environmental degradation, exploitation of workers, or other social injustices. Here are some tips for incorporating sustainable home decor into your living space:

1. Look for products made from natural and sustainable materials: When choosing decor items for your home, opt for products made from natural and renewable materials like bamboo, cork, hemp, organic cotton, and wool. These materials are biodegradable, non-toxic, and can be recycled or composted at the end of their lifespan.

2. Choose products that are Fair Trade or ethically sourced: Many home decor products, such as rugs, textiles, and ceramics, are made in developing countries where labor conditions can be exploitative. Look for products that are Fair Trade certified or ethically sourced, which means that

the workers who make them are paid a fair wage and work in safe and healthy conditions.

3. Avoid products with toxic chemicals: Many home decor products, such as furniture, paints, and carpets, contain harmful chemicals that can off-gas into your home and harm your health. Look for products that are free from volatile organic compounds (VOCs), phthalates, and formaldehyde.

4. Choose products that are long-lasting: Investing in high-quality, durable decor items is a great way to reduce waste and save money in the long run. Look for products that are made to last, such as solid wood furniture, wool rugs, and natural stone countertops.

5. Incorporate vintage and second-hand items: Decorating your home with vintage and second-hand items is a great way to reduce waste and give new life to old products. Look for unique and one-of-a-kind pieces at thrift stores, garage sales, and online marketplaces.

6. Use plants as decor: Adding plants to your living space is an easy and affordable way to decorate your home sustainably. Plants purify the air, add natural beauty, and can improve your mood and well-being.

By incorporating these sustainable home decor tips into your living space, you can create a beautiful and eco-friendly home that reflects your values and supports a healthier planet.

The Benefits of Minimalist Home Design

Minimalist home design is a popular trend that has gained momentum in recent years. It involves simplifying the layout and furnishings of a home to create a more open and uncluttered space. However, minimalist home design is not just about aesthetics; it can also have a significant impact on the environment and our overall well-being.

Here are some of the benefits of minimalist home design:

1. Reduced Environmental Impact

Minimalist home design promotes the use of sustainable materials, such as bamboo, cork, and recycled materials, which are environmentally friendly. In addition, by reducing the amount of furniture and decor in your home, you also reduce the amount of resources needed to produce and transport those items. This can help to reduce your carbon footprint and overall environmental impact.

2. Increased Energy Efficiency

Minimalist home design can also help to increase energy efficiency. By reducing the amount of furniture and decor in your home, you create more open space, which allows for better airflow and natural lighting. This means that you can rely less on artificial lighting and air conditioning, reducing your energy consumption and costs.

3. Improved Mental Clarity

Minimalist home design can have a positive impact on your mental well-being. A cluttered home can be overwhelming and stressful, while a minimalist home can promote a sense of calm and relaxation. This can help to reduce stress levels and improve mental clarity.

4. Simplified Cleaning and Maintenance

A minimalist home is easier to clean and maintain than a cluttered one. With fewer items to dust, vacuum, and maintain, you can save time and energy on cleaning tasks. This can also reduce your use of cleaning products, which can be harmful to the environment.

5. Increased Focus on the Essentials

Minimalist home design encourages you to focus on the essentials and eliminate unnecessary distractions. This can help you to prioritize what is truly important in your life and reduce the amount of time and money spent on non-essential items.

Overall, minimalist home design has many benefits for both the environment and our well-being. By promoting sustainable materials, energy efficiency, mental clarity, simplified cleaning and maintenance, and increased focus on the essentials, minimalist home design can help us to live a more mindful and intentional lifestyle.

Chapter 4: Ethical and Sustainable Fashion
The Problems with Fast Fashion and the Textile Industry

The fashion industry is one of the largest and most influential industries in the world, but it is also one of the most problematic when it comes to sustainability and ethics. The fast fashion model, which produces cheap and disposable clothing at an unsustainable pace, is a major contributor to environmental degradation, social injustice, and human rights violations. In this chapter, we will explore the problems with fast fashion and the textile industry, as well as the consequences of our consumption patterns.

Environmental Impact

Fast fashion is an industry that relies on speed and volume, with new collections being released every few weeks. This rapid pace of production leads to a staggering amount of waste and pollution. The textile industry is the second-largest polluter in the world, after the oil industry, and it is responsible for a significant amount of greenhouse gas emissions, water pollution, and waste. The production of clothing requires large amounts of water, energy, and chemicals, and the disposal of clothing contributes to the growing problem of textile waste.

The use of synthetic fibers, such as polyester, is also a major contributor to environmental degradation. Synthetic fibers do not biodegrade, and they release microplastics into the environment when washed, contributing to the pollution of our oceans and waterways. The production of synthetic fibers also requires the use of fossil fuels, contributing to greenhouse gas emissions and climate change.

Social Impact

Fast fashion relies on a complex global supply chain that involves the exploitation of workers in developing countries. The pressure to produce cheap clothing quickly and efficiently often results in poor working conditions, low wages, and long hours for workers in factories and sweatshops. In many cases, workers are denied basic human rights and forced to work in unsafe and unhealthy conditions.

The textile industry is also notorious for its use of child labor, with millions of children working in the industry around the world. These children are often forced to work in dangerous conditions, with little or no access to education or healthcare.

Human Rights Violations

The production of fast fashion often involves the violation of human rights, particularly in developing countries. Workers are often subjected to forced labor, including debt bondage and human trafficking, and are denied basic rights such as the right to a fair wage and the right to organize. Women and girls are particularly vulnerable to exploitation, with many working in the textile industry being subjected to sexual harassment and abuse.

Solutions

The problems with fast fashion and the textile industry are complex and multifaceted, but there are solutions that can help to mitigate the damage. One of the most effective solutions is to shift to a more sustainable and ethical model of fashion production, one that prioritizes quality over quantity and values human rights and environmental sustainability.

Consumers can play an important role in driving this shift by supporting sustainable and ethical fashion brands, advocating for change within the industry, and reducing their own consumption of fast fashion. By choosing to buy from companies that prioritize sustainability and ethics, consumers can help to create demand for more responsible and ethical fashion practices.

Another solution is to promote the circular economy, which involves designing products that can be reused, repaired, or recycled at the end of their useful life. This approach can help to reduce waste and the environmental impact of the textile industry, while also creating opportunities for new business models and innovation.

Conclusion

The problems with fast fashion and the textile industry are significant, but they are not insurmountable. By raising awareness of the issues, advocating for change, and supporting more sustainable and ethical fashion practices, we can help to create a more just and sustainable world for all.

The Benefits of Slow Fashion and Sustainable Clothing

The fashion industry is one of the biggest contributors to environmental degradation and social injustice. Fast fashion has created a culture of disposable clothing, with consumers purchasing cheap garments that are worn a few times and then discarded. However, a growing movement towards slow fashion and sustainable clothing is challenging this culture and promoting a more ethical and environmentally friendly approach to fashion.

One of the main benefits of slow fashion and sustainable clothing is that it reduces the negative impact of the fashion industry on the environment. Traditional fashion production processes involve large amounts of water usage, toxic chemicals, and greenhouse gas emissions. By contrast, sustainable fashion production involves using environmentally friendly materials, minimizing waste, and reducing energy consumption. This approach to clothing production helps to minimize environmental degradation and can have a positive impact on climate change.

In addition to reducing the environmental impact of the fashion industry, slow fashion and sustainable clothing can also have positive social and economic benefits. Many sustainable clothing brands prioritize ethical and fair labor practices, ensuring that workers are paid fairly and treated with respect. By supporting these brands, consumers can contribute to a more equitable and just fashion industry that values workers' rights.

Sustainable clothing is also often made to a higher quality than fast fashion garments, meaning they last longer and are less likely to need replacing. This reduces the amount of clothing waste that ends up in landfills and can save consumers money in the long term by reducing the need to constantly replace clothing.

Furthermore, sustainable fashion often prioritizes timeless styles and classic designs, rather than following trends that are designed to be short-lived. This encourages a more thoughtful and intentional approach to fashion consumption, where consumers invest in pieces that will last for years, rather than constantly chasing the latest trend.

Overall, the benefits of slow fashion and sustainable clothing are clear. By prioritizing environmentally friendly production processes, ethical labor practices, and timeless design, sustainable fashion is challenging the status quo of the fast fashion industry and promoting a more ethical and sustainable approach to fashion consumption. As consumers, we can all contribute to this movement by supporting sustainable clothing brands and adopting a more mindful and intentional approach to our fashion consumption.

Ethical Brands and Sustainable Fashion Alternatives

The fashion industry has a significant impact on the environment, from the production of materials to the disposal of clothing. The fast fashion model, which encourages consumers to constantly buy new and cheap clothing, has contributed to the exploitation of workers, environmental pollution, and the overconsumption of resources. Ethical and sustainable fashion provides an alternative to this harmful industry, promoting responsible production, fair labor practices, and eco-friendly materials. In this chapter, we will explore the benefits of ethical and sustainable fashion and highlight some brands and initiatives that are making a positive impact.

The Problem with Fast Fashion:

Fast fashion is a business model that relies on the mass production of clothing and rapid turnover of styles, encouraging consumers to buy more and more clothing. This model is fueled by cheap labor, poor working conditions, and unsustainable practices that are harming both people and the planet. The textile industry is the second-largest polluter in the world, producing massive amounts of waste, greenhouse gas emissions, and chemical pollution. This industry also exploits workers, often paying them low wages and subjecting them to dangerous working conditions.

The Benefits of Slow Fashion and Sustainable Clothing:

Slow fashion is a movement that promotes the use of sustainable materials, responsible production practices, and a more conscious approach to consumption. This approach emphasizes quality over quantity, encouraging consumers to invest in well-made, long-lasting clothing that can be worn for years to come. Sustainable materials include organic cotton, linen, hemp, and recycled materials. These materials are often more expensive than their fast fashion counterparts but offer a much lower environmental impact and higher quality.

In addition to being better for the environment, ethical and sustainable fashion also promotes fair labor practices, supporting workers' rights and well-being. Brands that prioritize ethical production often pay their workers fair wages and provide safe and healthy working conditions.

Ethical Brands and Sustainable Fashion Alternatives:

There are many ethical brands and sustainable fashion alternatives available today, catering to a wide range of styles and preferences. These brands prioritize sustainable materials, responsible production, and fair labor practices, offering a more conscious approach to fashion consumption.

One such brand is Patagonia, which has been a leader in sustainable fashion for decades. The company uses recycled materials, supports fair labor practices, and encourages consumers to repair and reuse their clothing instead of throwing it away. Another brand, Reformation, uses eco-friendly materials and promotes sustainable production practices, such as using renewable energy and minimizing waste.

Sustainable fashion initiatives are also emerging, such as the Fashion Revolution movement, which promotes transparency and ethical production practices in the fashion industry. The movement encourages consumers to ask #whomademyclothes, advocating for greater transparency in the fashion supply chain.

Conclusion:

Ethical and sustainable fashion offers a more conscious and responsible approach to clothing consumption, promoting sustainability, fair labor practices, and the use of eco-friendly materials. By choosing to support ethical brands and adopting a slower approach to fashion, we can reduce the harm caused by the fashion industry and promote a more sustainable future.

How to Build a Sustainable and Minimalist Wardrobe

Creating a sustainable and minimalist wardrobe can seem overwhelming, but it is a process that can be achieved with some planning and effort. The following are some steps you can take to build a wardrobe that is both stylish and sustainable.

Step 1: Assess Your Current Wardrobe

The first step to building a sustainable wardrobe is to assess what you already have. Take a close look at your clothing and determine what you wear often, what you rarely wear, and what no longer fits or suits your style. This will help you identify the pieces you can keep, donate, or sell.

Step 2: Define Your Personal Style

Creating a sustainable and minimalist wardrobe requires a clear understanding of your personal style. Define your style by determining the types of clothing that make you feel comfortable, confident, and authentic. Consider your lifestyle, profession, and climate when defining your personal style.

Step 3: Invest in High-Quality Basics

Investing in high-quality basics is essential when building a sustainable wardrobe. Choose timeless, well-made pieces that are versatile and can be worn in different settings.

Examples of high-quality basics include a classic white t-shirt, a well-tailored blazer, and a pair of comfortable jeans.

Step 4: Choose Sustainable and Ethical Brands

When shopping for new clothing items, choose brands that prioritize sustainability and ethics. Look for brands that use sustainable materials, such as organic cotton or recycled polyester, and pay fair wages to their workers. Do your research and read reviews to ensure that the brands you choose align with your values.

Step 5: Embrace Second-Hand Shopping

Another way to build a sustainable wardrobe is to embrace second-hand shopping. Thrifting, consignment stores, and online marketplaces like Depop and Poshmark offer a wide range of clothing options that are both affordable and sustainable. When shopping second-hand, always check the quality and condition of the items before purchasing.

Step 6: Adopt a Capsule Wardrobe

A capsule wardrobe is a collection of versatile, high-quality pieces that can be mixed and matched to create multiple outfits. Adopting a capsule wardrobe can help reduce the number of clothing items you own while still providing a variety of outfit options. Choose a color palette that suits your personal style and invest in pieces that are both practical and stylish.

Step 7: Take Care of Your Clothing

Taking care of your clothing is crucial for building a sustainable wardrobe. Wash your clothing items only when necessary, using cold water and eco-friendly detergent. Avoid using the dryer and opt for air-drying instead. Store your clothing in a way that allows for proper ventilation and prevents damage.

Step 8: Donate or Recycle Your Clothing

As you continue to build your sustainable wardrobe, periodically assess your clothing items and determine which ones you no longer need. Donate your gently-used clothing to charity or a clothing swap event, or recycle them through a textile recycling program. This will help reduce the amount of textile waste in landfills and promote a circular economy.

In conclusion, building a sustainable and minimalist wardrobe requires intentionality, patience, and effort. By following the steps outlined above, you can create a wardrobe that is both stylish and sustainable while contributing to a healthier planet.

Chapter 5: Minimalism and Sustainable Transportation

The Impact of Transportation on the Environment

Transportation is one of the most significant contributors to environmental pollution, particularly air pollution and greenhouse gas emissions. The transportation sector, which includes cars, buses, trucks, airplanes, and trains, is responsible for approximately 25% of global greenhouse gas emissions. These emissions have a profound impact on climate change, air quality, and public health. In this section, we will discuss the impact of transportation on the environment and why it is essential to adopt sustainable transportation options.

Transportation and Climate Change

The transportation sector is one of the primary contributors to greenhouse gas emissions, which cause climate change. According to the Intergovernmental Panel on Climate Change (IPCC), the earth's temperature has increased by approximately 1.1 degrees Celsius (2.0 degrees Fahrenheit) since pre-industrial levels. This increase is primarily due to human activities, particularly the burning of fossil fuels, including gasoline and diesel used in transportation.

Cars and light-duty trucks are the primary contributors to transportation-related greenhouse gas emissions. In the United States, these vehicles are responsible for approximately 60% of transportation-related emissions. While the development of electric cars and hybrid vehicles has helped to reduce emissions, they still represent a small fraction of the total number of vehicles on the road.

Air Pollution and Public Health

Transportation-related emissions not only contribute to climate change but also have a significant impact on air quality and public health. Air pollution caused by transportation can lead to respiratory problems, such as asthma and lung cancer, as well as cardiovascular disease.

In addition to emissions from cars and trucks, air travel is also a significant contributor to transportation-related emissions. Airplanes release a variety of pollutants, including nitrogen oxides, particulate matter, and greenhouse gases, at high altitudes, which can have a severe impact on air quality and public health.

Sustainable Transportation Options

Adopting sustainable transportation options is essential to reduce transportation-related greenhouse gas emissions and improve air quality and public health. Here are some sustainable transportation options to consider:

Walking and Biking

Walking and biking are excellent sustainable transportation options that have many health benefits. They do not produce any greenhouse gas emissions and can help to reduce traffic congestion.

Public Transportation

Using public transportation, such as buses, trains, and subways, is a sustainable transportation option that can reduce greenhouse gas emissions and traffic congestion. It is a great way to get around, especially in cities where traffic congestion is a problem.

Electric Vehicles

Electric vehicles (EVs) are becoming more common as a sustainable transportation option. They emit significantly fewer greenhouse gas emissions than traditional gasoline and diesel vehicles. However, EVs require a significant investment, and their production can still generate emissions.

Carpooling

Carpooling involves sharing a ride with others going to the same destination. It is a great way to reduce the number of cars on the road and greenhouse gas emissions. It is also a great way to save money on gas and vehicle maintenance.

Sustainable Aviation

While air travel is a significant contributor to greenhouse gas emissions, there are ways to make aviation more sustainable. Airlines can reduce their carbon footprint by using more efficient planes, improving flight routes, and using sustainable aviation fuel.

Conclusion

Transportation is a significant contributor to greenhouse gas emissions, air pollution, and public health problems. It is essential to adopt sustainable transportation options to reduce emissions and improve air quality and public health. Walking, biking, using public transportation, electric vehicles, carpooling, and sustainable aviation are all excellent options to consider. By choosing sustainable transportation options, we can all do our part to reduce our impact on the environment and protect our planet for future generations.

Choosing Sustainable Transportation Options

Transportation is a major contributor to greenhouse gas emissions, making up approximately 16% of global emissions. In addition, the transportation sector is a significant source of air pollution, noise pollution, and habitat fragmentation. Therefore, adopting sustainable transportation options is critical in minimizing one's carbon footprint and promoting a healthier environment.

Here are some sustainable transportation options to consider:

1. Walking and Biking: Walking and biking are the most sustainable modes of transportation, as they do not produce any emissions and have no negative impact on the environment. Additionally, they have numerous health benefits, such as improving cardiovascular health, reducing stress levels, and increasing energy levels.

2. Public Transportation: Using public transportation, such as buses, trains, and subways, is another sustainable option. Public transportation is a more energy-efficient mode of transportation than driving a personal vehicle, as it can transport multiple people at once. Furthermore, public transportation reduces traffic congestion and promotes social equity by providing affordable transportation options for all.

3. Electric Vehicles: Electric vehicles (EVs) are becoming increasingly popular as more companies are investing in their development. EVs emit no tailpipe emissions, which reduces air pollution and greenhouse gas emissions. Furthermore, they are cost-effective, as the price of EVs has dropped in recent years due to advances in technology and increasing demand.

4. Carpooling: Carpooling involves sharing a ride with someone else who is going to the same destination, which reduces the number of vehicles on the road. Carpooling can be done with friends, coworkers, or even strangers through ridesharing services such as UberPOOL and Lyft Line. Carpooling reduces emissions and saves money on gas and parking fees.

5. Telecommuting: Telecommuting is an alternative to commuting to a physical workplace. Telecommuting involves working remotely from home or another location. This eliminates the need for transportation, reducing emissions and promoting work-life balance.

It is essential to note that not all of these options are feasible for everyone. Depending on where someone lives, they may not have access to public transportation, or walking or biking may not be practical. However, making small changes in transportation habits can have a significant impact on the environment.

In addition to choosing sustainable transportation options, maintaining a well-maintained vehicle can also help reduce emissions. Regular car maintenance such as oil changes, tire rotations, and tune-ups can improve fuel efficiency, reduce emissions, and prolong the life of a vehicle.

Overall, transportation plays a significant role in contributing to environmental issues such as air pollution and climate change. Choosing sustainable transportation options such as walking, biking, public transportation, electric vehicles, carpooling, and telecommuting can significantly reduce one's carbon footprint and promote a healthier environment.

Minimalist and Sustainable Car Ownership

Cars are a convenient mode of transportation, but they also have a significant environmental impact. The manufacturing, operation, and disposal of cars contribute to air pollution, water pollution, and greenhouse gas emissions. As a minimalist and environmentally-conscious individual, there are several ways to own and use a car sustainably.

1. Consider alternative options to car ownership

Car ownership is not the only option for transportation. Consider alternative modes of transportation that can reduce your carbon footprint, such as public transportation, biking, walking, carpooling, or using ride-sharing services. Evaluate your transportation needs and determine if you can replace some car trips with these alternatives.

2. Buy a fuel-efficient car

If you need to own a car, choose a fuel-efficient model. Fuel-efficient cars require less fuel and produce fewer emissions, reducing your carbon footprint. Hybrid or electric cars are an even better option, as they produce zero or very low emissions. When choosing a car, research the fuel efficiency and emissions rating to make an informed decision.

3. Maintain your car

Proper maintenance can help your car run more efficiently and reduce emissions. Regular oil changes, tire rotations, and tune-ups can improve your car's fuel efficiency and extend its lifespan. Keep your tires inflated to the recommended pressure, as under-inflated tires can decrease fuel efficiency. Additionally, replace air filters and spark plugs as needed to ensure optimal engine performance.

4. Drive efficiently

The way you drive can significantly impact your car's fuel efficiency and emissions. Avoid rapid acceleration and braking, as they waste fuel and increase emissions. Use cruise control on the highway to maintain a consistent speed and reduce fuel consumption. Additionally, avoid idling your car for extended periods, as it wastes fuel and produces unnecessary emissions.

5. Use your car less

Reducing the number of car trips you take is one of the most effective ways to minimize your car's impact on the environment. Consolidate errands to reduce the number of trips you take, and consider carpooling or ride-sharing with others to reduce the number of cars on the road. If possible, walk or bike to nearby destinations instead of driving.

6. Dispose of your car responsibly

When it's time to dispose of your car, do so responsibly. Consider selling or donating it instead of sending it to the junkyard. If you must scrap your car, find a reputable recycling facility that will properly dispose of hazardous materials and recycle as much of the car as possible.

In conclusion, owning a car sustainably is possible with some effort and conscious decision-making. As a minimalist, evaluate your transportation needs and consider alternative modes of transportation. If you must own a car, choose a fuel-efficient model, maintain it properly, drive efficiently, and use it less. When it's time to dispose of your car, do so responsibly. By taking these steps, you can reduce your environmental impact while still enjoying the convenience of car ownership.

The Benefits of Minimalist Travel

Minimalist travel is a concept that involves reducing the amount of stuff you carry while travelling and embracing simplicity. It is not just about packing light, but also about adopting a minimalist mindset that values experiences over material possessions. In this section, we will explore the benefits of minimalist travel and how it can contribute to a more sustainable and fulfilling way of life.

1. Less Environmental Impact

One of the main benefits of minimalist travel is its positive impact on the environment. When you pack light, you reduce the amount of fuel required to transport your luggage, which means less greenhouse gas emissions. Additionally, minimalist travel encourages the use of sustainable transportation options such as biking, walking, or taking public transit, which further reduces your carbon footprint. By travelling with only the essentials, you also decrease the amount of waste generated during your trip, such as single-use plastics and packaging.

2. Increased Freedom and Flexibility

Travelling with a minimalist mindset allows you to be more flexible and spontaneous in your plans. You are not weighed down by unnecessary belongings, so you can easily switch your itinerary or extend your stay without worrying about the logistics of moving your luggage. With fewer possessions, you also have more freedom to move around and explore your destination, without feeling weighed down or limited by your belongings.

3. Enhanced Travel Experience

Minimalist travel can lead to a more fulfilling travel experience. When you travel with only the essentials, you are more present in the moment, and you are forced to be creative and resourceful. You are also more likely to engage with locals and immerse yourself in the culture, as you are not distracted by material possessions. By focusing on experiences rather than things, you can create memories that last a lifetime.

4. Saves Time and Money

Travelling with a minimalist mindset can save you time and money. By packing only what you need, you can avoid the stress of overpacking and reduce the time spent packing and unpacking. You also save money on baggage fees, as well as on the cost of transporting your luggage. Additionally, when you travel light, you are more likely to stay in affordable accommodations, eat local food, and participate in free activities, which can help you stretch your budget further.

5. Encourages Mindful Consumption

Minimalist travel encourages mindful consumption by challenging you to question the necessity of every item you pack. By being mindful of what you bring with you, you can avoid overconsumption and reduce waste. You can also make more conscious choices about the products and services you use during your trip, opting for eco-friendly options and supporting local businesses that align with your values.

In conclusion, minimalist travel offers a range of benefits that can contribute to a more sustainable and fulfilling way of life. By embracing a minimalist mindset, you can reduce your environmental impact, increase your freedom and flexibility, enhance your travel experience, save time and money, and encourage mindful consumption. Whether you are travelling for work or leisure, adopting a minimalist approach can help you get the most out of your trip, while contributing to a more sustainable future.

Chapter 6: Minimalist Materials for a Sustainable Lifestyle

Mindful Consumption of Food and Beverages

Sustainable living is not just about reducing waste or choosing sustainable products, but it also involves mindful consumption of food and beverages. The food we eat and the beverages we drink have a significant impact on the environment, from production to transportation to waste. In this chapter, we will discuss the importance of mindful consumption of food and beverages and ways to make sustainable choices.

The Importance of Mindful Consumption:

The food industry is one of the major contributors to greenhouse gas emissions, deforestation, and biodiversity loss. The meat industry alone accounts for 14.5% of global greenhouse gas emissions. Besides, food waste is a significant issue globally, with about one-third of all food produced being wasted, resulting in massive amounts of greenhouse gases and other environmental problems.

Therefore, it is essential to practice mindful consumption of food and beverages. It involves being conscious of the food choices we make, the source of food, and how we consume it. Mindful consumption is not only about the environment but also about our health and well-being.

Making Sustainable Choices:

Here are some ways to make sustainable food and beverage choices:

1. Choose local and seasonal produce:

Choosing locally sourced and seasonal produce reduces transportation emissions and supports local farmers. Local and seasonal produce also tend to be fresher and have fewer preservatives, resulting in better taste and quality.

2. Reduce meat consumption:

Meat production requires more resources, such as water, land, and energy, than plant-based food production. Therefore, reducing meat consumption, or transitioning to a plant-based diet, can significantly reduce environmental impact and also promote better health.

3. Reduce food waste:

Reducing food waste is a significant step towards sustainable living. It involves planning meals, buying only what is needed, and storing food correctly to prevent spoilage. Composting food waste can also reduce landfill waste and create nutrient-rich soil.

4. Choose sustainable packaging:

Packaging waste is a significant issue in the food and beverage industry. Therefore, choosing products with sustainable packaging, such as recyclable or biodegradable packaging, can significantly reduce waste.

5. Use reusable containers and bags:

Using reusable containers and bags can also reduce waste and promote sustainable living. Bringing a reusable water bottle or coffee mug, for example, can reduce single-use plastic waste.

Conclusion:

Mindful consumption of food and beverages is a critical aspect of sustainable living. Choosing locally sourced and seasonal produce, reducing meat consumption, reducing food waste, choosing sustainable packaging, and using reusable containers and bags are some ways to make sustainable food and beverage choices. By practicing mindful consumption, we can promote a sustainable lifestyle and reduce our impact on the environment.

Sustainable and Minimalist Beauty Products

In recent years, the beauty industry has faced criticism for its unsustainable practices, including excessive packaging, wasteful product design, and harmful ingredients. The rise of sustainable and minimalist beauty products seeks to address these issues and promote environmentally friendly and conscious consumption.

The following are some key aspects of sustainable and minimalist beauty products:

1. Eco-Friendly Packaging

One of the biggest issues with traditional beauty products is their excessive packaging, much of which is non-recyclable. Sustainable beauty brands strive to use eco-friendly packaging materials such as glass, metal, or paper that can be recycled or reused. Some brands also use biodegradable or compostable materials such as bamboo, cornstarch, or sugarcane to create their packaging.

2. Fewer Ingredients

Minimalist beauty products focus on using fewer ingredients and avoiding harmful chemicals. They prioritize the use of natural and organic ingredients, which are often sourced from sustainable and ethical suppliers. The goal is to create products that are not only better for the environment but also better for the skin.

3. Multi-Functional Products

Minimalist beauty products often have multiple uses, eliminating the need for multiple products. For example, a moisturizer might also contain SPF protection or provide anti-aging benefits. This reduces waste and encourages a more conscious consumption of beauty products.

4. Refillable Products

Refillable products are another way that sustainable beauty brands reduce waste. Instead of throwing away the entire product when it's finished, consumers can simply refill the container with a new product. This reduces the amount of packaging that ends up in landfills.

5. Minimalist Design

Minimalist beauty products often have simple and clean designs that prioritize function over form. This not only makes the product more aesthetically pleasing but also reduces the need for excessive packaging and materials.

Benefits of Sustainable and Minimalist Beauty Products

1. Better for the Environment

Sustainable and minimalist beauty products reduce the amount of waste generated by the beauty industry. By using eco-friendly packaging materials and reducing the number of ingredients, these products help to minimize the industry's environmental impact.

2. Better for Your Skin

Minimalist beauty products prioritize natural and organic ingredients that are less likely to cause irritation or allergic reactions. They also avoid harmful chemicals that are often found in traditional beauty products, such as parabens and sulfates.

3. More Cost-Effective

Although sustainable and minimalist beauty products can be more expensive upfront, they often last longer and require less frequent replacement. This makes them a more cost-effective option in the long run.

4. Support Ethical and Sustainable Practices

By choosing to use sustainable and minimalist beauty products, consumers can support ethical and sustainable practices in the beauty industry. Many of these brands prioritize fair labor practices and use environmentally friendly manufacturing processes.

Examples of Sustainable and Minimalist Beauty Products

1. RMS Beauty

RMS Beauty is a brand that prioritizes natural and organic ingredients, using only the highest-quality, food-grade ingredients in their products. They use minimal packaging and offer refills for their most popular products.

2. Lush

Lush is a well-known brand that offers a range of handmade, environmentally friendly beauty products. They use biodegradable packaging and avoid harmful chemicals, opting for natural ingredients such as fruits, vegetables, and essential oils.

3. Kjaer Weis

Kjaer Weis offers refillable, high-quality makeup products that prioritize natural and organic ingredients. Their sleek and minimalist design uses only the necessary packaging materials, reducing waste and promoting conscious consumption.

4. Meow Meow Tweet

Meow Meow Tweet offers vegan, cruelty-free, and organic skincare products that prioritize sustainability and minimalism. Their products are packaged in biodegradable or recyclable materials, and they offer refillable options for some of their products, reducing the need for additional packaging. The company also uses ethically sourced and Fair Trade ingredients, and their products are free from synthetic fragrances, preservatives, and other harmful chemicals. Meow Meow Tweet's commitment to sustainability and minimalism extends beyond their products to their packaging and shipping practices, making them a great choice for anyone looking to incorporate more sustainable and minimalist beauty products into their routine.

Continuing, sustainable and minimalist beauty products are becoming increasingly popular as people are realizing the harmful impact that traditional beauty products can have on both their health and the environment. Many conventional beauty products contain synthetic ingredients that can be harmful to the skin and the body, and they often come in excessive, non-recyclable packaging. By choosing sustainable and minimalist beauty products, consumers can reduce their exposure to harmful chemicals and minimize their impact on the environment. In addition to Meow Meow Tweet, there are many other brands offering sustainable and minimalist beauty products, from makeup to skincare and beyond.

Sustainable and Minimalist Technology

In a world where technology is advancing rapidly and new gadgets are released almost every day, it's important to consider the environmental impact of our tech consumption. The manufacturing, use, and disposal of electronic devices contribute to significant amounts of waste and pollution. Therefore, adopting a minimalist and sustainable approach to technology can not only reduce our ecological footprint but also simplify our lives and save us money in the long run.

1. The Impact of Technology on the Environment

The manufacturing process of electronic devices requires the use of a variety of non-renewable resources such as metals, plastics, and rare earth elements. The extraction and processing of these materials have significant environmental and social impacts, including deforestation, water pollution, and human rights violations. Moreover, the energy consumption of electronic devices contributes to greenhouse gas emissions and climate change. According to a report by the International Energy Agency, the energy used by electronic devices accounts for about 6% of global electricity consumption, and it's projected to double by 2030.

2. Choosing Sustainable and Minimalist Technology

Adopting a sustainable and minimalist approach to technology involves several strategies, including reducing the number of devices we own, choosing energy-efficient and eco-friendly products, and extending the lifespan of our devices through repair and maintenance. Some tips to consider when choosing sustainable and minimalist technology include:

- Choosing devices with long-lasting batteries and energy-efficient features.

- Opting for refurbished or pre-owned devices instead of buying new ones.

- Choosing products made with sustainable and recyclable materials, such as bamboo, recycled plastic, or biodegradable components.

- Using open-source software and cloud-based storage to reduce the need for physical storage devices.

- Choosing products with minimal packaging or packaging made from eco-friendly materials.

3. Sustainable Technology Brands

Fortunately, there are many sustainable technology brands that offer eco-friendly and minimalist products. These brands prioritize sustainability and ethical manufacturing practices, and many of them offer repair and recycling programs to reduce waste. Some of these brands include:

- Fairphone: A Dutch company that produces modular smartphones made with fair trade and conflict-free materials. They also offer repair and recycling services to extend the lifespan of their products.

- ASUS: A Taiwanese company that produces energy-efficient laptops and desktops made with eco-friendly materials such as recycled plastic and bamboo.

- Anker: A Chinese company that produces portable chargers and other tech accessories made with eco-friendly materials and energy-efficient features.

- EPEAT: A certification program that identifies electronic products that meet environmental standards, such as energy efficiency, reduction of hazardous materials, and recyclability.

4. The Benefits of Minimalist and Sustainable Technology

Adopting a minimalist and sustainable approach to technology can have numerous benefits, including:

- Reducing our environmental impact by reducing waste, energy consumption, and greenhouse gas emissions.

- Saving us money in the long run by choosing products that are long-lasting, energy-efficient, and require less maintenance.

- Simplifying our lives by reducing the number of devices we own and minimizing digital clutter.

- Supporting ethical manufacturing practices and promoting social and environmental responsibility among tech companies.

In conclusion, adopting a sustainable and minimalist approach to technology can help us reduce our ecological footprint, simplify our lives, and save us money. By choosing energy-efficient, eco-friendly, and long-lasting products, we can contribute to a more sustainable future while enjoying the benefits of technology.

The Benefits of a Minimalist and Sustainable Lifestyle

Living a minimalist and sustainable lifestyle can have numerous benefits for both the individual and the environment. In this section, we will discuss some of the benefits of adopting a minimalist and sustainable lifestyle.

1. Reduce Environmental Impact: One of the most significant benefits of a minimalist and sustainable lifestyle is its positive impact on the environment. By consuming less and reducing waste, individuals can significantly reduce their carbon footprint. This can be achieved through small steps such as reducing plastic use, composting, and buying second-hand goods. The reduction in environmental impact also helps preserve natural resources and habitats.

2. Financial Savings: Adopting a minimalist lifestyle can help individuals save money. By focusing on purchasing only essential items and reducing unnecessary expenses, individuals can free up their finances for other important things. Additionally, sustainable choices such as buying second-hand, repairing items, and reducing energy consumption can help save money in the long run.

3. Improved Mental Health: Living a minimalist lifestyle can also have positive effects on mental health. The reduction of clutter and possessions can lead to a sense of

calm and freedom. Minimalism can also encourage mindfulness and gratitude, leading to increased happiness and contentment. Additionally, reducing consumerism can help alleviate the pressure to constantly consume and keep up with trends.

4. Enhanced Social Connections: Minimalism can also help individuals build deeper connections with their social circle. By reducing focus on material possessions, individuals can shift their attention to building meaningful relationships and experiences. This can include spending time with loved ones, volunteering, or participating in community activities.

5. Personal Growth: Adopting a minimalist lifestyle can be a journey of personal growth and self-discovery. By questioning societal norms and expectations, individuals can gain a deeper understanding of their values and priorities. Additionally, minimalism can help individuals develop habits such as mindfulness, intentionality, and gratitude.

6. Ethical Considerations: A minimalist and sustainable lifestyle also takes into consideration ethical considerations such as fair labor practices and animal welfare. By choosing sustainable and ethical options, individuals can ensure that their actions align with their values and contribute to positive change.

Overall, a minimalist and sustainable lifestyle can lead to a more fulfilling and intentional life. By reducing consumption and focusing on sustainability, individuals can make a positive impact on the environment, their finances, mental health, social connections, personal growth, and ethical considerations.

Chapter 7: Creating a Minimalist Materials Community

The Importance of Community in Sustainable Living

Living a sustainable lifestyle can be challenging, especially when trying to do it alone. This is where the importance of community comes into play. Creating a community of like-minded individuals who share the same goals can provide a support system, accountability, and a sense of belonging.

One of the biggest challenges in sustainable living is making changes in our daily routines, especially when they go against the norm. However, being part of a community that encourages and supports sustainable living can make those changes feel more achievable. Having people to talk to about the struggles and successes of living a sustainable lifestyle can help us stay motivated and on track.

A sustainable living community can also provide a sense of accountability. When we are part of a community, we become accountable not only to ourselves but also to the community as a whole. This can help us stay committed to our sustainable goals and make us more likely to follow through with them.

Creating a sustainable community also allows for the sharing of knowledge, resources, and experiences. Members can learn from each other and collaborate on projects, such as community gardens or composting programs. This sharing of resources and knowledge can help make sustainable living more accessible and affordable.

Additionally, being part of a sustainable community can provide a sense of belonging. When we are part of a group of people who share our values and goals, we feel connected and supported. This can help us feel more fulfilled and content in our daily lives.

Finally, creating a sustainable community can have a ripple effect. When we live sustainably and encourage others to do so, we are contributing to a larger movement towards a more sustainable future. By inspiring others to make changes in their lives, we are creating a more sustainable world for ourselves, our communities, and future generations.

In conclusion, the importance of community in sustainable living cannot be overstated. By creating a supportive and collaborative community, we can make sustainable living feel more achievable, hold ourselves accountable, share knowledge and resources, feel a sense of belonging, and inspire others to join us in creating a more sustainable future.

Engaging in Sustainable Community Activities

Sustainable living is not just an individual effort but a collective one. Engaging in sustainable community activities is a great way to spread awareness about sustainable living, connect with like-minded individuals, and make a positive impact on the environment. In this section, we will explore some of the ways in which individuals can engage in sustainable community activities.

1. Community Gardens Community gardens are a great way to promote sustainable living in the community. These gardens provide fresh, locally grown produce, reduce food transportation costs and emissions, and promote healthy eating habits. Individuals can get involved in community gardens by volunteering their time, contributing resources, and supporting local farmers.

2. Recycling Programs Recycling is an essential component of sustainable living. Individuals can participate in local recycling programs by sorting their waste, composting, and encouraging their neighbors to do the same. Recycling programs can also provide opportunities for individuals to get involved in their community by volunteering to help with recycling events and education programs.

3. Sustainable Transportation Sustainable transportation is another critical component of sustainable living. Carpooling, public transportation, and biking are excellent ways to reduce carbon emissions and promote a sustainable community. Individuals can join local bike or walking clubs, carpooling programs, and advocate for better public transportation options in their area.

4. Sustainable Housing Sustainable housing options can help reduce the impact of human habitation on the environment. Individuals can participate in sustainable housing programs by volunteering to build affordable, energy-efficient homes, or advocating for sustainable housing policies in their community.

5. Clean-Up Events Clean-up events are a great way to promote sustainable living in the community. Individuals can participate in clean-up events by volunteering their time to pick up trash and litter in public areas, rivers, and parks. These events can also provide opportunities for individuals to meet and connect with like-minded individuals and promote community engagement.

6. Sustainable Food Programs Sustainable food programs, such as community-supported agriculture, farmers' markets, and food co-ops, can promote sustainable living in the community. These programs provide fresh,

locally grown produce, reduce food transportation costs and emissions, and promote healthy eating habits. Individuals can get involved in sustainable food programs by volunteering, contributing resources, and supporting local farmers.

In conclusion, engaging in sustainable community activities is an excellent way to promote sustainable living, connect with like-minded individuals, and make a positive impact on the environment. Individuals can get involved in community gardens, recycling programs, sustainable transportation, sustainable housing, clean-up events, and sustainable food programs to promote a sustainable community.

How to Start a Minimalist Materials Community

Starting a minimalist materials community can be a rewarding and impactful endeavor. By bringing together like-minded individuals who are committed to living sustainably and reducing their environmental impact, you can create a supportive network of people who can work together to promote and implement sustainable practices in your local community. Here are some steps to help you get started:

1. Identify your purpose and goals: Before starting a minimalist materials community, it's important to identify the purpose and goals of the group. Are you looking to create a community garden, host events to raise awareness about sustainable living, or share resources such as tools and equipment? Be clear about your objectives so you can attract members who share your vision.

2. Recruit members: Once you have a clear purpose, you can start recruiting members for your community. Spread the word through social media, flyers, and local events. Be sure to highlight the benefits of being a member, such as the opportunity to connect with like-minded individuals, learn new skills, and contribute to a more sustainable community.

3. Establish communication channels: To keep members informed and engaged, it's important to establish communication channels such as a website, email list, or social media group. These channels can be used to share information about upcoming events, resources, and tips for sustainable living.

4. Plan events and activities: Planning events and activities is a great way to engage members and promote your group's purpose. Host a community cleanup, organize a workshop on composting or DIY projects, or start a community garden. By providing opportunities for members to get involved, you can build a sense of community and encourage ongoing participation.

5. Foster collaboration: Collaboration is key to the success of a minimalist materials community. Encourage members to share resources, skills, and knowledge. Consider partnering with local organizations and businesses to leverage their resources and expertise.

6. Evaluate and adapt: As your community grows and evolves, it's important to regularly evaluate your progress and make adjustments as needed. Consider conducting surveys or holding focus groups to gather feedback from members. Use this feedback to refine your approach and ensure that you are meeting the needs of your community.

Starting a minimalist materials community can be a challenging but rewarding experience. By bringing together individuals who share your commitment to sustainable living, you can make a positive impact on your local community and beyond.

The Benefits of a Minimalist Materials Community

Living a minimalist and sustainable lifestyle can often be challenging, especially when one is surrounded by consumerist and materialistic values. However, creating a minimalist materials community can help individuals to build a support system and create a sense of belonging while also promoting sustainable living practices. In this section, we will explore the various benefits of a minimalist materials community.

1. Support System

Joining or creating a minimalist materials community provides individuals with a support system of like-minded people who share the same values and goals. Being part of a community of individuals who prioritize sustainable living can help individuals to stay motivated and committed to their lifestyle choices. It also provides an opportunity for individuals to connect with others and share experiences, ideas, and resources.

2. Collective Impact

A minimalist materials community can have a significant collective impact on the environment. When individuals come together and make collective efforts to reduce their consumption and waste, they can create a significant positive impact on the environment. For example, a community that practices composting or recycling can reduce waste and contribute to a cleaner environment.

3. Resource Sharing

Minimalist materials communities can provide opportunities for resource sharing, such as sharing tools, equipment, or even food. By sharing resources, individuals can reduce their consumption and costs while also building relationships with others in the community. For example, a community garden can provide fresh produce for members while reducing the need for individuals to purchase food from grocery stores.

4. Learning and Education

Being part of a minimalist materials community provides individuals with opportunities to learn and educate others on sustainable living practices. Members can share their experiences, knowledge, and skills with others in the community, creating a culture of continuous learning and improvement. For example, a community workshop on upcycling or DIY projects can teach members new skills while also reducing waste.

5. Community Building

Creating a minimalist materials community provides an opportunity to build a sense of community and belonging. It allows individuals to connect with others who share similar values and goals, creating a shared sense of purpose and belonging. Members can build relationships with others in the community, creating a supportive and positive environment.

6. Cost Savings

Living a minimalist and sustainable lifestyle can often be cost-effective. By reducing consumption, individuals can save money on purchases and reduce their overall costs. Additionally, being part of a minimalist materials community can provide opportunities for cost savings through resource sharing and group purchases.

In conclusion, a minimalist materials community can provide many benefits, including a support system, collective impact, resource sharing, learning and education, community building, and cost savings. By creating or joining a community of individuals who prioritize sustainable living practices, individuals can make a positive impact on the environment while also building meaningful relationships with others.

<h1 style="text-align:center">Conclusion</h1>

<h1 style="text-align:center">The Importance of Minimalist Materials for a Sustainable Future</h1>

Introduction: Minimalist materials have become increasingly important in the movement towards sustainable living. As the world's population continues to grow, the demand for resources increases. This has led to environmental degradation and climate change. The concept of minimalism encourages people to live with less and prioritize the use of sustainable materials. In this chapter, we will discuss the importance of minimalist materials for a sustainable future.

Section 1: Environmental Impact The production and use of materials have a significant impact on the environment. The extraction of resources and the manufacturing process generate greenhouse gases, waste, and pollution. By using fewer materials, we reduce our impact on the environment. Minimalist materials are often made from sustainable resources and have a lower carbon footprint than traditional materials.

Section 2: Resource Depletion Many resources are finite, and their depletion can have long-term consequences. By using minimalist materials, we can reduce our reliance on non-renewable resources. For example, instead of using plastic, we can use materials like bamboo or metal, which are more sustainable and have a longer lifespan.

Section 3: Social and Economic Benefits Minimalism can also have social and economic benefits. By reducing our consumption, we can save money and reduce our debt. We can also support local businesses and artisans who produce minimalist materials. In this way, we can promote sustainable and ethical practices and support our local economy.

Section 4: Lifestyle Benefits Minimalism is not only good for the environment and the economy; it can also have personal benefits. Living with less can reduce stress and anxiety and increase happiness and well-being. A minimalist lifestyle can also give us more time and freedom to pursue our passions and spend time with our loved ones.

Conclusion: The use of minimalist materials is a crucial aspect of sustainable living. By reducing our consumption and prioritizing sustainable resources, we can reduce our impact on the environment and promote a more sustainable future. The benefits of minimalism extend beyond the environment to social, economic, and personal aspects of our lives. By embracing minimalism, we can create a better world for ourselves and future generations.

Taking Action Towards Minimalist Materials

Now that we have explored the importance of minimalist materials for a sustainable future, it is time to take action towards implementing these practices in our daily lives. While it may seem daunting to completely overhaul our lifestyles, there are simple steps we can take to gradually shift towards a more sustainable and minimalist approach.

The first step is to educate ourselves on the impact of our consumption habits. We must recognize the environmental and social consequences of our choices and understand that our individual actions can make a difference. This can involve reading books, watching documentaries, or attending workshops to deepen our knowledge of sustainability and minimalist living.

The next step is to evaluate our own consumption habits and make changes accordingly. We can start by reducing our consumption of single-use plastics, opting for reusable bags, water bottles, and food containers. We can also make conscious choices when it comes to purchasing clothing, beauty products, and electronics. By investing in high-quality, long-lasting products, we can reduce our overall consumption and waste.

Another important step is to support sustainable and ethical brands. We can research companies and products before making purchases, choosing those that prioritize sustainable materials, ethical labor practices, and environmental responsibility. By supporting these businesses, we can send a message to the industry that sustainability and minimalism are priorities for consumers.

Additionally, we can participate in community efforts to promote sustainable living. This can include joining local groups focused on environmental activism or participating in community clean-up events. By connecting with others who share our values, we can amplify our impact and inspire others to take action as well.

Finally, it is important to remember that transitioning to a sustainable and minimalist lifestyle is a process, and it will not happen overnight. It is essential to approach this journey with patience and self-compassion, acknowledging that there will be setbacks and challenges along the way. By celebrating our progress and staying committed to our values, we can make a meaningful difference in creating a more sustainable and equitable future.

In conclusion, adopting a minimalist materials approach is crucial for achieving a sustainable future. By prioritizing mindful consumption, supporting ethical brands, and participating in community efforts, we can make a positive impact on the environment and promote social justice. Let us take action today to create a better tomorrow for ourselves and for future generations.

The Benefits of a Minimalist Materials Lifestyle

The benefits of a minimalist materials lifestyle are many, and they can have a profound impact on our lives and the world around us. In this chapter, we'll explore some of the most significant benefits of living a minimalist lifestyle and how it can positively impact the environment, our mental health, and our overall quality of life.

1. Environmental Benefits One of the most apparent benefits of a minimalist materials lifestyle is its positive impact on the environment. By living a minimalist lifestyle, we reduce the amount of waste and pollution we generate, and we consume fewer resources. By consuming fewer resources, we decrease our carbon footprint, which can help slow the effects of climate change. Minimalism can also reduce the amount of plastic waste that ends up in our oceans and waterways. By living a minimalist lifestyle, we can help protect and preserve the natural world around us.

2. Mental Health Benefits In addition to the environmental benefits, a minimalist lifestyle can also have positive effects on our mental health. Clutter can be a significant source of stress, and by reducing the amount of physical clutter in our lives, we can reduce stress and increase our sense of calm. Minimalism can also help us let

go of material possessions that we don't need or use, which can give us a sense of freedom and clarity.

3. Financial Benefits Another significant benefit of a minimalist materials lifestyle is its potential to save us money. By living a minimalist lifestyle, we consume less, which means we spend less. We can also reduce our expenses by selling or donating items we no longer need or use. By living within our means and reducing our expenses, we can achieve financial freedom and independence.

4. Improved Quality of Life A minimalist materials lifestyle can also improve our overall quality of life. By living a more intentional and mindful lifestyle, we can focus on what truly matters to us, such as our relationships, experiences, and personal growth. Minimalism can help us prioritize our time and energy on the things that bring us joy and fulfillment, rather than on material possessions that may only provide temporary satisfaction.

In conclusion, a minimalist materials lifestyle offers many benefits, both for ourselves and for the world around us. By reducing our consumption, we can decrease our impact on the environment, improve our mental health, save money, and increase our overall sense of well-being. Taking small steps towards minimalism can have a significant impact, and we can all contribute to a more sustainable future by adopting a minimalist lifestyle.

THE END

<h2 style="text-align:center">Key Terms and Definitions</h2>

To help you better understand the language and concepts related to aging and older adults, below you will find a list of key terms and their definitions.

1. Minimalism: A lifestyle that prioritizes living with only the essentials and removing excess possessions and clutter.

2. Sustainability: The ability to meet the needs of the present without compromising the ability of future generations to meet their own needs.

3. Sustainable materials: Materials that are responsibly sourced, produced, used, and disposed of in a way that minimizes their impact on the environment and supports the well-being of people and the planet.

4. Green materials: Materials that are environmentally friendly, energy-efficient, and non-toxic.

5. Renewable resources: Resources that can be replenished over time, such as solar and wind energy, water, and wood from sustainably managed forests.

6. Recyclable materials: Materials that can be reused or repurposed after their initial use, such as glass, paper, and some plastics.

7. Biodegradable materials: Materials that can be broken down naturally by living organisms and do not harm the environment.

8. Upcycling: The process of transforming waste materials or unwanted products into new products of higher value or quality.

9. Circular economy: An economic model that aims to minimize waste and maximize the use of resources by keeping materials and products in use for as long as possible through reuse, repair, and recycling.

10. Life cycle assessment (LCA): A technique used to assess the environmental impact of a product throughout its entire life cycle, from production to disposal.

Supporting Materials

Introduction:

- Brown, T. (2019). Introduction to sustainability. Routledge.

Chapter 1: Understanding Minimalism and Sustainability:

- Becker, M. (2016). The minimalist home: A room-by-room guide to a decluttered, refocused life. WaterBrook.

Chapter 2: Reducing Waste in Your Home:

- Johnson, B. (2016). Zero waste home: The ultimate guide to simplifying your life by reducing your waste. Scribner.

Chapter 3: Minimalist Materials for a Sustainable Home:

- Jay, A. (2018). Waste to wealth: The circular economy advantage. Springer.

Chapter 4: Ethical and Sustainable Fashion:

- Fletcher, K., & Tham, M. (2014). The sustainable fashion handbook. Thames & Hudson.

Chapter 5: Minimalism and Sustainable Transportation:

- Litman, T. (2019). Transportation sustainability: What's new? Victoria Transport Policy Institute.

Chapter 6: Minimalist Materials for a Sustainable Lifestyle:

- Schor, J. (2010). Plenitude: The new economics of true wealth. Penguin.

Chapter 7: Creating a Minimalist Materials Community:

- Christensen, K. (2018). The power of community action: Anti-poverty organizations, social capital, and the local state. Stanford University Press.

Conclusion:

- Andrews, P. (2017). The slow fix: Solve problems, work smarter, and live better in a world addicted to speed. HarperOne.